NURSING ESSENTIALS

A Nurse Comprehensive Guide to Core Competencies

Clara Henderson

Table of Contents

Chapter 1: Foundations of Nursing Competencies

Introduction... 5

The Evolution of Nursing: Historical
Perspectives and Modern Roles.................. 10

The Nursing Process: A Framework for
Competent Care... 14

Chapter 2: Clinical Assessment and Skills

Health Assessment: Mastering the Art of
Patient Evaluation.......................................19

Vital Signs Monitoring: Foundations of
Patient Care.. 23

Medication Administration: Safely and
Accurately Administering Medications.......28

Infection Control: Ensuring Patient and
Healthcare Worker Safety...........................34

Wound Care: Principles and Best Practices.39

Chapter 3: Critical Thinking and Decision-Making

Clinical Reasoning: Developing Critical Thinking Skills............................. 45

Diagnostic Testing: Interpreting Results and Clinical Implications.................................. 51

Emergency Preparedness: Responding Swiftly and Effectively...............................57

Chapter 4: Effective Communication

Therapeutic Communication: Building Trusting Patient Relationships.....................63

Family-Centered Care: Engaging and Supporting Patients' Loved Ones................ 68

Interprofessional Collaboration: Working Effectively in Healthcare Teams.................72

Chapter 5: Ethical Practice and Cultural Competence

Nursing Ethics: Navigating Complex Moral

Issues.. 78

Legal Aspects of Nursing: Understanding the
Legal Framework...................................... 83

Cultural Competence: Providing Culturally
Sensitive Care...88

Chapter 6: Education and Patient Advocacy

Patient Education: Empowering Patients for
Self-Care...93

Palliative and End-of-Life Care: Ensuring
Comfort and Dignity.................................. 98

Healthcare Quality Improvement:
Implementing Evidence-Based Practice....103

Chapter 7: Leadership and Management

Leadership in Nursing: Influencing Positive
Change...109

Healthcare Management: Navigating
Administrative Roles............................... 114

Professional Development: Advancing Your
Nursing Career...119

Chapter 8: Safety and Regulation

Patient Safety: Preventing Errors and
Adverse Events...125

Regulatory Compliance: Upholding Nursing
Standards.. 130

Conclusion: Mastering Nursing Essentials

Embracing Lifelong Learning: Thriving as a
Competent Nurse..................................... 136

Chapter 1:
Foundations of Nursing Competencies

Introduction

Nursing is a noble and dynamic profession that plays a pivotal role in healthcare systems worldwide. It's a profession that demands not only compassion and dedication but also a high level of competence. Nursing is the art and science of caring for individuals, families, and communities, and its effectiveness hinges on nurses' ability to possess and continually develop a set of core competencies.

Each chapter in "Nursing Essentials" provides in-depth insights, practical guidance, and real-life examples to help nurses develop and enhance their core competencies. This comprehensive guide serves as an invaluable resource for nursing students, educators, and practicing nurses seeking to excel in their roles and deliver high-quality care to patients across diverse healthcare settings.

In this introductory chapter, we embark on a journey into the heart of nursing practice by defining and exploring these core competencies. These competencies are the foundation upon which nursing care is built, and they encompass a wide array of knowledge, skills, and attributes that nurses must possess to provide safe, effective, and patient-centered care.

The Evolution of Nursing Competencies

Nursing as a profession has evolved significantly over the years. From Florence Nightingale's pioneering work in the 19th century to the complex, multidisciplinary healthcare environment of today, nursing competencies have adapted to meet the changing needs of patients and the healthcare system.

Early in nursing's history, the focus was primarily on providing basic care and comfort. However, as medical knowledge expanded and healthcare became more sophisticated, the role of the nurse evolved. Today, nurses are not only caregivers but also educators, advocates, leaders, and researchers.

The Nursing Process: A Framework for Competent Care

At the core of nursing competencies lies the nursing process, a systematic framework that guides nurses in delivering patient-centered care. The nursing process consists of five key steps: assessment, diagnosis, planning, implementation, and evaluation. Each of these steps requires a distinct set of competencies.

Assessment: Nurses must be skilled in gathering comprehensive patient information, including health history, physical assessment findings, and psychosocial data.

Diagnosis: Competent nurses can identify and prioritize patient needs based on their assessment findings and nursing diagnoses.

Planning: Planning involves setting specific goals and developing a care plan tailored to each patient's unique needs.

Implementation: Nurses implement the care plan, delivering interventions and treatments while maintaining safety and adherence to best practices.

Evaluation: Competency in evaluation entails the ability to assess the effectiveness of interventions, make necessary adjustments, and document outcomes.

The Essence of Nursing Competencies

Nursing competencies encompass a wide range of skills and attributes, including clinical expertise, critical thinking, effective communication, ethical practice, and cultural competence. These competencies enable nurses to provide holistic care that addresses not only the physical aspects of health but also the emotional, social, and cultural dimensions.

As you embark on your journey through this comprehensive guide on nursing essentials, you will delve deeper into each competency, gaining insights and practical knowledge that will help you excel in your nursing practice. Whether you are a nursing student, an educator, or a practicing nurse, this guide will serve as a valuable resource to refine your competencies, enhance your patient care, and contribute to the noble profession of nursing.

The Evolution of Nursing: Historical Perspectives and Modern Roles

Nursing is a profession deeply rooted in history, and its evolution over the centuries has been both remarkable and essential to the development of modern healthcare. In this part, we embark on a journey through time to explore the historical perspectives of nursing and how these foundations have shaped the multifaceted roles of modern nurses.

The origins of nursing can be traced back to ancient civilizations. In ancient Egypt, Greece, and Rome, individuals known as "healers" or "caregivers" provided rudimentary medical care and comfort to the sick. Often, these early caregivers were women, and their role was closely tied to their familial and communal duties.

The true transformation of nursing into a respected profession can be attributed to Florence Nightingale, a British nurse who is often considered the founder of modern nursing. During the Crimean War in the mid-19th century, Nightingale and her team of nurses provided exceptional care to wounded soldiers. Her meticulous record-keeping and emphasis on hygiene and sanitation revolutionized healthcare practices.

The Evolution of Nursing Education

As nursing gained recognition as a profession, nursing education became formalized. Nursing schools were established, and curricula expanded to include anatomy, physiology, and clinical training. The shift from an apprenticeship model to structured education elevated the standards of nursing care.

Today's nurses play diverse and crucial roles in healthcare. They are caregivers, educators, advocates, leaders, and researchers. Modern nurses work in various healthcare settings, including hospitals, clinics, schools, and community organizations. They provide care to patients across the lifespan, from newborns to the elderly, and across a spectrum of specialties, from pediatrics to critical care.

Specialization and Advanced Practice

Nursing has also seen the emergence of specialized roles and advanced practice. Nurse practitioners, nurse anesthetists, nurse midwives, and clinical nurse specialists have expanded their scope of practice, providing a broader range of healthcare services. These advanced practitioners often work independently and collaborate closely with physicians to deliver comprehensive care.

Challenges and Opportunities in Modern Nursing

While nursing has made tremendous progress, it also faces contemporary challenges. These include workforce shortages, burnout, and the ever-evolving landscape of healthcare technology and regulations. However, with these challenges come opportunities for innovation, leadership, and the continued improvement of patient care.

The Ongoing Legacy of Nursing

The evolution of nursing from its humble beginnings to its current multifaceted roles is a testament to the resilience, dedication, and adaptability of nurses throughout history. As we move forward, nursing remains at the forefront of healthcare, adapting to new challenges, embracing technology, and advocating for the well-being of patients and communities. Understanding this historical journey helps us appreciate the vital role that nurses play in shaping the future of healthcare.

The Nursing Process: A Framework for Competent Care

The nursing process is the cornerstone of nursing practice, providing a systematic and holistic approach to delivering competent and patient-centered care. In this part, we delve into the nursing process as a dynamic framework that guides nurses in assessing, diagnosing, planning, implementing, and evaluating care. Understanding and mastering the nursing process is essential for nurses at all levels of practice.

Assessment: The Foundation of Care

The first step in the nursing process is assessment. Nurses systematically collect data from patients through interviews, physical examinations, and reviewing medical records. This holistic assessment considers not only the patient's physical health but also their psychological, social, and cultural aspects. Effective assessment informs the nurse about the patient's needs, strengths, and potential risks.

Diagnosis: Identifying Patient Needs

Based on the assessment data, nurses make nursing diagnoses. These are distinct from medical diagnoses and focus on actual or potential health problems that nursing care can address. Nursing diagnoses guide the planning and implementation of patient-centered interventions.

Planning: Developing a Care Plan

Planning involves setting goals and creating a care plan tailored to the patient's unique needs. Nursing care plans outline interventions, timelines, and expected outcomes. They serve as roadmaps for nursing care delivery and help nurses prioritize care and ensure that interventions are evidence-based and patient-focused.

Implementation: Providing Patient-Centered Care

Implementation is the stage where nursing interventions are put into action. Nurses administer medications, perform procedures, provide education, and coordinate care with other healthcare team members. Effective communication and documentation are crucial during this phase to ensure continuity of care and patient safety.

Evaluation: Assessing the Effectiveness of Interventions

Evaluation is an ongoing process throughout the patient's care journey. Nurses continually assess the patient's response to interventions and compare the outcomes to the goals set in the care plan. If outcomes are not met, nurses modify the plan and interventions as needed. This iterative process ensures that care remains patient-centered and responsive to changing needs.

The Iterative Nature of the Nursing Process

It's important to recognize that the nursing process is iterative, meaning it can cycle back to previous stages as new information becomes available or as the patient's condition changes. This adaptability allows nurses to provide responsive and patient-focused care.

Enhancing Critical Thinking and Decision-Making

The nursing process is a tool that enhances critical thinking and decision-making in nursing practice. It empowers nurses to make informed clinical judgments, prioritize care, and advocate for patients' needs. Critical thinking is a core competency that nurses continually develop throughout their careers.

The Nursing Process in Action

The nursing process is not a linear, one-size-fits-all approach but rather a dynamic framework that adapts to the unique needs of each patient. As nurses engage with this process, they provide competent, evidence-based, and patient-centered care. Understanding the nursing process and honing the skills associated with each stage is fundamental to nursing practice and the delivery of high-quality healthcare.

Chapter 2:
Clinical Assessment and Skills

Health Assessment: Mastering the Art of Patient Evaluation

Health assessment is a foundational skill in nursing that involves the systematic collection and analysis of patient data to inform clinical decision-making and provide comprehensive care. In this chapter, we explore the art and science of health assessment, emphasizing its significance in nursing practice and patient outcomes.

The Importance of Health Assessment

Health assessment is often the first step in the nursing process and serves as a crucial starting point for understanding a patient's health status. It involves gathering data on various aspects of a patient's physical, psychological, and social well-being. This information forms the basis for nursing diagnoses, care planning, and interventions.

Holistic Assessment: Seeing the Whole Patient

A hallmark of nursing health assessment is its holistic nature. Nurses consider not only the physical aspects of health but also the patient's emotional, social, cultural, and spiritual dimensions. This comprehensive approach recognizes that health is influenced by a multitude of factors beyond just bodily functions.

Types of Health Assessment

Health assessment can be broadly categorized into two types:

Comprehensive Assessment: This involves a detailed examination of all body systems and is typically conducted upon admission to a healthcare facility or during routine check-ups. It establishes a baseline for ongoing care.

Focused Assessment: Focused assessments target specific body systems or areas of concern. They are often performed in response to changes in a patient's condition or to address particular health issues.

The Health History Interview

One of the key components of health assessment is the health history interview. During this conversation with the patient, nurses gather information about the patient's medical history, current health concerns, lifestyle, and psychosocial factors. Effective communication and active listening are crucial in obtaining accurate and relevant information.

Physical Examination Skills

In addition to health history, physical examination skills are fundamental to health assessment. Nurses use techniques such as inspection, palpation, percussion, and auscultation to gather data about the patient's body systems. Thorough and systematic examination ensures that no important findings are missed.

Documentation and Critical Thinking

Accurate and timely documentation of assessment findings is vital for continuity of care and communication among healthcare team members. Nurses also employ critical thinking skills to interpret the data they collect, identify potential health problems, and make clinical judgments.

Cultural Competence in Health Assessment

Cultural competence is essential in health assessment to ensure that care is respectful and sensitive to the patient's cultural background and beliefs. Effective cross-cultural communication and understanding are vital in gathering relevant data.

The Art and Skill of Health Assessment

Health assessment is not just a routine task; it is an art that requires sensitivity, empathy, and a keen eye for detail, as well as a skill that must be continually refined and updated. As nurses master the art of health assessment, they empower themselves to provide holistic, patient-centered care that addresses the unique needs and circumstances of each individual under their care.

Vital Signs Monitoring: Foundations of Patient Care

Vital signs monitoring is a fundamental aspect of patient care in healthcare settings. It involves the regular measurement and assessment of vital signs, which are essential physiological indicators of a patient's overall health and well-being. In this part, we explore the significance of vital signs monitoring as a foundational element of patient care.

Understanding Vital Signs

Vital signs are a set of objective measurements that provide critical information about a patient's physiological status. The four primary vital signs are:

Body Temperature: Body temperature is a measure of the body's internal heat. It helps identify fever, hypothermia, or hyperthermia, which can be indicative of various health conditions.

Pulse Rate (Heart Rate): Pulse rate is the number of heartbeats per minute. It reflects the heart's pumping efficiency and can indicate cardiac function, circulation, and response to stress.

Respiratory Rate: Respiratory rate is the number of breaths a patient takes per minute. It helps assess the adequacy of ventilation and can reveal respiratory distress or dysfunction.

Blood Pressure: Blood pressure measures the force of blood against the walls of arteries. It consists of two values: systolic (the pressure during a heartbeat) and diastolic (the pressure between heartbeats). Blood pressure provides insight into cardiovascular health and perfusion.

The Role of Vital Signs in Patient Care

Vital signs serve several critical roles in patient care:

Early Detection of Health Changes: Vital signs are often the first indicators of a patient's deteriorating health. Monitoring them regularly can help identify issues early, allowing for prompt intervention.

Assessment of Treatment Effectiveness: Changes in vital signs can reflect how a patient is responding to treatment. For instance, a fever may decrease with antipyretic medication, or blood pressure may stabilize with antihypertensive therapy.

Baseline Establishment: Initial vital sign measurements establish a baseline against which subsequent measurements are compared. This baseline aids in tracking a patient's progress or detecting deviations from their normal values.

Safety: Monitoring vital signs is crucial in critical care settings and during surgery to ensure patient safety and to detect complications promptly.

Techniques for Measuring Vital Signs

Healthcare professionals use various methods and instruments to measure vital signs, including:

- Thermometers for temperature measurement.
- Pulse oximeters to assess oxygen saturation in the blood.
- Stethoscopes to listen to heart and lung sounds.
- Blood pressure cuffs and sphygmomanometers to measure blood pressure.
- Observation of chest rise and fall for respiratory rate assessment.

Documentation and Communication

Accurate documentation of vital signs is essential for maintaining a patient's medical record and communicating vital information to the healthcare team. Timely and precise documentation ensures that changes in vital signs are promptly addressed, reducing the risk of adverse events.

The Backbone of Patient Care

Vital signs monitoring is the backbone of patient care, providing valuable insights into a patient's health status and guiding clinical decision-making. Nurses and healthcare professionals must be proficient in accurately measuring, interpreting, and documenting vital signs to provide safe and effective care. Regular monitoring of vital signs enhances patient safety, facilitates early intervention, and contributes to positive healthcare outcomes.

Medication Administration: Safely and Accurately Administering Medications

Medication administration is a critical aspect of nursing practice that requires precision, attention to detail, and a deep commitment to patient safety. We will explore the significance of safely and accurately administering medications in healthcare settings.

The Importance of Medication Administration

Medications are powerful tools in healthcare, offering the potential to treat, manage, or alleviate a wide range of health conditions. However, their effectiveness hinges on the safe and precise administration by healthcare professionals. Proper medication administration is vital for several reasons:

Patient Well-Being: Accurate medication administration directly impacts a patient's health and well-being. It can relieve pain, control chronic conditions, and save lives.

Avoiding Harm: Incorrect administration or dosage errors can lead to adverse drug reactions, side effects, or harm to patients. Preventing such errors is a paramount concern.

Legal and Ethical Obligations: Nurses are legally and ethically bound to administer medications safely and accurately. Deviations from medication protocols can have serious legal consequences.

Patient Education: Nurses often play a crucial role in educating patients about their medications, including how and when to take them and potential side effects.

Components of Medication Administration

Safe and accurate medication administration encompasses several critical components:

Assessment: Before administering any medication, nurses must assess the patient's medical history, allergies, current medications, and overall health status. This assessment helps identify potential contraindications or interactions.

Medication Orders: Nurses must have a valid and up-to-date medication order from a licensed prescriber. The order should specify the medication name, dosage, route of administration, frequency, and any other relevant instructions.

Patient Identification: Properly identifying the patient is crucial to ensure that the right medication is given to the right individual. Many healthcare facilities use multiple patient identifiers, such as name and date of birth, to verify identity.

Medication Preparation: Preparing medications accurately involves calculating the correct dosage, verifying the medication against the order, and using proper techniques for medication administration (e.g., sterile technique for injections).

Administration Route: Medications can be administered through various routes, including oral (by mouth), intravenous (IV), intramuscular (IM), subcutaneous (SubQ), and topical. Nurses must follow the prescribed route meticulously.

Documentation: Timely and accurate documentation of medication administration is essential. This includes recording the medication administered, dose, route, time, and any observed patient responses.

Preventing Medication Errors

Medication errors are a significant concern in healthcare. Nurses must adhere to best practices and strategies to prevent errors, such as the "Five Rights" of medication administration:

Right Patient: Verify the patient's identity before administering any medication.

Right Medication: Confirm that the medication matches the order and is appropriate for the patient.

Right Dose: Calculate and administer the correct dosage.

Right Route: Administer the medication through the prescribed route.

Right Time: Administer medications at the prescribed time or within the appropriate time window.

A Pillar of Patient Care

Medication administration is a pillar of patient care, requiring diligence, competence, and a commitment to patient safety. Nurses must continuously update their knowledge of medications, stay alert to potential drug interactions or allergies, and meticulously follow established protocols to ensure that each patient receives the right medication, in the right dose, through the right route, at the right time. Safe and accurate medication administration contributes significantly to positive patient outcomes and overall healthcare quality.

Infection Control: Ensuring Patient and Healthcare Worker Safety

Infection control is a paramount aspect of healthcare that focuses on preventing the spread of infections within healthcare settings, safeguarding both patients and healthcare workers. Let us delve into the critical importance of infection control in healthcare and the strategies employed to maintain a safe and sterile environment.

The Significance of Infection Control

Infections acquired within healthcare settings, often referred to as healthcare-associated infections (HAIs) or nosocomial infections, pose a significant threat to patients and healthcare workers.

Infection control is essential for several reasons:

Patient Safety: Infections can lead to severe complications, prolonged hospital stays, and, in some cases, fatalities. Preventing infections ensures the safety and well-being of patients.

Healthcare Worker Safety: Healthcare workers are also at risk of acquiring infections from patients. Infection control measures protect the occupational health of healthcare providers.

Cost Savings: HAIs result in substantial healthcare costs, including additional treatments, longer hospital stays, and increased use of resources. Infection control efforts help reduce these economic burdens.

Key Principles of Infection Control

Infection control in healthcare is guided by a set of fundamental principles:

Hand Hygiene: Hand hygiene is the single most important measure to prevent the spread of infections. Healthcare workers must practice proper handwashing or use hand sanitizers before and after patient contact.

Personal Protective Equipment (PPE): The appropriate use of PPE, such as gloves, masks, gowns, and eye protection, is essential when caring for patients with known or suspected infections.

Isolation Precautions: Isolation precautions, including contact, droplet, and airborne precautions, are used to prevent the transmission of specific pathogens. These precautions dictate the type of PPE and the level of isolation required.

Environmental Cleaning: Regular and thorough cleaning and disinfection of patient care areas, surfaces, and equipment are essential to prevent the transmission of infections.

Safe Injection Practices: Healthcare workers must follow safe injection practices to prevent the contamination of needles, syringes, and medication vials.

Respiratory Hygiene and Cough Etiquette: Patients and healthcare workers should practice respiratory hygiene, including covering coughs and sneezes, to reduce the spread of respiratory infections.

Antibiotic Stewardship: Appropriate and judicious use of antibiotics helps prevent antibiotic-resistant infections.

Infection Control in the Era of Infectious Diseases

Infection control has gained heightened importance in the face of infectious disease outbreaks, such as the COVID-19 pandemic. Healthcare facilities have implemented additional measures, including strict visitor policies, enhanced personal protective equipment requirements, and isolation protocols, to contain the spread of infectious agents.

Education and Training

Education and training are vital components of infection control. Healthcare workers must receive regular training on infection prevention practices, including proper hand hygiene, the use of PPE, and adherence to isolation precautions. Ongoing education ensures that healthcare providers remain up-to-date with the latest guidelines and best practices.

Protecting Health and Well-Being

Infection control is a cornerstone of modern healthcare, aimed at protecting the health and well-being of both patients and healthcare workers. Effective infection control measures, when rigorously implemented, reduce the risk of healthcare-associated infections and contribute to safer, more effective healthcare delivery.

Wound Care: Principles and Best Practices

Wound care is a critical component of healthcare that focuses on the assessment, treatment, and management of wounds to facilitate the healing process and prevent complications. In this part, we explore the principles and best practices of wound care, highlighting its significance in patient recovery and overall well-being.

The Importance of Wound Care

Wounds can result from various causes, including surgical procedures, injuries, chronic medical conditions, and accidents.

Proper wound care is essential for several reasons:

Facilitating Healing: Effective wound care promotes the body's natural healing processes, allowing tissues to repair and regenerate.

Preventing Infections: Wounds are susceptible to infections, which can lead to complications and delayed healing. Appropriate wound care reduces the risk of infection.

Minimizing Scarring: Properly managed wounds are less likely to develop excessive scarring or other cosmetic concerns.

Pain Management: Adequate wound care helps manage pain and discomfort associated with wounds.

Key Principles of Wound Care

Wound care is guided by a set of fundamental principles:

Assessment: The first step in wound care is a thorough assessment of the wound. This includes evaluating the wound's size, depth, type, location, and any signs of infection or inflammation. A comprehensive assessment guides treatment decisions.

Infection Control: Preventing and treating wound infections are paramount. This involves keeping the wound clean, using sterile techniques, and administering antibiotics when necessary.

Debridement: Removing dead or damaged tissue from the wound (debridement) is often necessary to promote healing. Debridement can be surgical, mechanical, enzymatic, or autolytic, depending on the wound's characteristics.

Moist Wound Healing: Maintaining a moist wound environment is generally more conducive to healing than allowing wounds to dry out. Dressings and topical treatments help create this environment.

Protection and Support: Wounds need protection from further injury or contamination. Appropriate dressings, bandages, or splints are used to safeguard the wound.

Nutrition and Hydration: Proper nutrition and hydration are crucial for wound healing. Adequate protein, vitamins, and minerals are necessary for tissue repair.

Pain Management: Managing pain is an integral part of wound care. Healthcare providers may prescribe pain medications or use other pain management techniques, such as topical anesthetics.

Patient Education: Educating patients and caregivers about wound care is essential. This includes instructions on dressing changes, signs of complications, and when to seek medical attention.

Types of Wounds

Wounds come in various forms, including:

Acute Wounds: These result from injuries or surgical procedures and typically have well-defined edges.

Chronic Wounds: Chronic wounds, such as diabetic ulcers or pressure ulcers, often have delayed healing and may require specialized care.

Surgical Wounds: These result from surgical procedures and require meticulous care to prevent infection.

Burns: Burns are a specific type of wound that requires specialized assessment and management based on their depth and severity.

Advanced Wound Care

In some cases, advanced wound care techniques may be necessary. These include the use of advanced dressings, negative pressure wound therapy, and bioengineered skin substitutes.

Enhancing Healing and Well-Being

Wound care is a vital aspect of healthcare aimed at enhancing the healing process, preventing complications, and improving patients' quality of life. It demands a comprehensive understanding of wound assessment, infection control, and treatment principles. When performed with precision and adherence to best practices, wound care contributes significantly to patients' recovery and overall well-being.

Chapter 3:
Critical Thinking and Decision-Making

Clinical Reasoning: Developing Critical Thinking Skills

Clinical reasoning is a cognitive process that healthcare professionals, including nurses and physicians, use to make sense of patient information, analyze data, evaluate options, and arrive at clinical decisions. It's a core component of clinical practice and involves developing critical thinking skills. In this explanation, we explore clinical reasoning, its importance in healthcare, and how it fosters the development of critical thinking skills.

The Significance of Clinical Reasoning

Clinical reasoning serves as the bridge between theoretical knowledge and practical application in healthcare. It is crucial for several reasons:

Effective Patient Care: Clinical reasoning helps healthcare professionals make informed decisions about patient assessment, diagnosis, treatment, and care planning. This ensures that patients receive appropriate and individualized care.

Problem Solving: Clinical reasoning involves problem-solving, enabling healthcare providers to address complex and dynamic healthcare challenges.

Reducing Errors: Developing strong clinical reasoning skills reduces the likelihood of diagnostic errors, medication errors, and other adverse events.

Enhancing Communication: Effective clinical reasoning fosters better communication among healthcare team members, leading to coordinated and patient-centered care.

Continuous Learning: Clinical reasoning is a dynamic process that encourages lifelong learning and the integration of new evidence-based practices into clinical care.

Developing Critical Thinking Skills through Clinical Reasoning

Critical thinking is a fundamental component of clinical reasoning, and the two are closely intertwined. Here's how clinical reasoning contributes to the development of critical thinking skills:

Data Collection: Clinical reasoning begins with gathering patient data, including medical history, physical assessments, and diagnostic test results. Critical thinking skills are needed to select relevant data, differentiate between important and less important information, and recognize patterns or trends.

Analysis: Healthcare providers critically analyze data to identify potential issues, risks, or deviations from the norm. This involves comparing patient data to established norms and recognizing when further investigation is required.

Clinical Judgment: Clinical reasoning leads to clinical judgment, where healthcare professionals make decisions about patient care. Critical thinking skills are essential in weighing the pros and cons of different options and selecting the most appropriate course of action.

Reflection: After implementing a care plan, healthcare providers reflect on the outcomes and evaluate their decisions. Critical thinking skills are necessary to assess the effectiveness of interventions and make adjustments as needed.

Problem-Solving: Clinical reasoning often involves addressing complex problems, such as diagnosing rare conditions or managing multiple comorbidities. Critical thinking skills enable healthcare professionals to tackle these challenges systematically and creatively.

Interprofessional Collaboration: Effective clinical reasoning supports collaboration with other healthcare team members. Critical thinking skills aid in communicating and understanding differing viewpoints, which is vital in team-based care.

Promoting Critical Thinking and Clinical Reasoning

Healthcare institutions and educational programs actively promote critical thinking and clinical reasoning through various means:

Education: Formal education, such as nursing and medical programs, incorporates critical thinking into the curriculum through problem-solving exercises, case studies, and discussions.

Simulation: Simulated clinical scenarios allow students and healthcare professionals to practice clinical reasoning in a controlled environment.

Continuing Education: Healthcare professionals engage in ongoing learning to stay updated with the latest research and evidence-based practices, which enhances their clinical reasoning abilities.

Mentorship: Experienced healthcare providers mentor students and junior colleagues, sharing their clinical reasoning processes and insights.

Peer Collaboration: Collaborative practice among peers encourages critical discussions and the exchange of ideas, fostering the development of critical thinking skills.

Nurturing Clinical Excellence

Clinical reasoning, rooted in critical thinking skills, is essential for providing high-quality healthcare. Developing these skills is a lifelong journey for healthcare professionals, and it contributes not only to improved patient outcomes but also to the continual advancement of healthcare practice.

Diagnostic Testing: Interpreting Results and Clinical Implications

Diagnostic testing plays a pivotal role in modern healthcare, aiding healthcare professionals in confirming or ruling out medical conditions, guiding treatment decisions, and monitoring patient progress. This part explores the significance of diagnostic testing, the process of interpreting test results, and their clinical implications.

The Significance of Diagnostic Testing

Diagnostic testing is essential in healthcare for several reasons:

Accurate Diagnosis: Testing helps healthcare providers accurately diagnose medical conditions, allowing for appropriate treatment planning.

Treatment Guidance: Diagnostic results guide treatment decisions, helping healthcare professionals choose the most effective interventions.

Disease Screening: Some tests are used for early disease detection, enabling timely intervention and improved outcomes.

Monitoring: Diagnostic tests are crucial for monitoring disease progression, treatment effectiveness, and patient recovery.

Interpreting Diagnostic Test Results

Interpreting diagnostic test results is a complex process that involves more than just reading numbers or values. It requires clinical judgment, an understanding of the test's sensitivity and specificity, consideration of patient history, and integration with other clinical information. The steps in interpreting test results include:

Understanding Reference Ranges: Most diagnostic tests have reference ranges that define what is considered normal for a particular population. Results falling within this range are typically considered normal, while those outside it may indicate a problem.

Clinical Context: Results must be interpreted in the context of the patient's clinical history, symptoms, and other diagnostic findings. A result that falls outside the reference range may not always indicate disease.

Sensitivity and Specificity: It's crucial to understand the sensitivity (the ability to detect true positives) and specificity (the ability to identify true negatives) of the test. A high false positive rate can lead to unnecessary anxiety and interventions, while a high false negative rate may result in missed diagnoses.

Repeat Testing: If a result is unexpected or inconclusive, healthcare providers may recommend repeat testing or additional tests to confirm or rule out a condition.

Consultation: In some cases, test results may be ambiguous or require expert interpretation. Healthcare providers may consult with specialists or pathologists for a more accurate assessment.

Clinical Implications of Diagnostic Results

The clinical implications of diagnostic test results vary widely based on the type of test and the condition being investigated. Some common clinical implications include:

Diagnosis Confirmation: Positive test results may confirm the presence of a specific medical condition, allowing for targeted treatment.

Disease Severity: Test results can provide insight into the severity of a disease, which may impact treatment decisions and prognosis.

Treatment Adjustment: In some cases, test results may necessitate adjustments to a patient's treatment plan, such as changing medications or dosages.

Prognosis: Diagnostic testing can help predict disease progression and long-term outcomes, assisting healthcare providers in providing appropriate patient counseling.

Monitoring: Many diagnostic tests are used for ongoing monitoring, allowing healthcare providers to assess treatment effectiveness and disease progression over time.

Screening: Some tests, like cancer screenings or prenatal testing, are used for early disease detection or risk assessment.

Patient Education

Patient education is a crucial component of the diagnostic testing process. Healthcare providers must communicate results clearly, explain their clinical implications, and address any questions or concerns patients may have. Patient understanding and involvement in decision-making are essential for optimal healthcare outcomes.

Guiding Care with Precision

Diagnostic testing is a cornerstone of modern healthcare, providing valuable information for disease diagnosis, treatment planning, and patient monitoring. Accurate interpretation of test results within the clinical context is essential to ensure that patients receive the most appropriate care, ultimately improving healthcare outcomes and patient well-being.

Emergency Preparedness: Responding Swiftly and Effectively

Emergency preparedness is a critical aspect of healthcare and public safety, involving proactive planning, training, and resources to respond swiftly and effectively to various emergencies, disasters, and crises. This part explores the importance of emergency preparedness, the key components of preparedness plans, and the principles of effective response.

The Importance of Emergency Preparedness

Emergency preparedness is vital for several reasons:

Life Preservation: It saves lives by ensuring that healthcare facilities, personnel, and resources are ready to respond to emergencies promptly and efficiently.

Injury Reduction: Preparedness measures can reduce the number and severity of injuries during emergencies.

Resource Allocation: Effective preparedness helps allocate resources where they are needed most efficiently, preventing shortages and ensuring that critical care is provided.

Community Resilience: Communities that are well-prepared for emergencies are more resilient and can recover faster from disasters.

Key Components of Emergency Preparedness

Risk Assessment: Identifying potential risks and hazards that may affect the healthcare facility and its community is the first step in preparedness planning.

Planning and Coordination: Developing comprehensive emergency plans that outline roles, responsibilities, communication strategies, and resource allocation is crucial.

Coordination with local, regional, and national agencies is also essential.

Training and Education: Healthcare personnel should receive regular training and education in emergency response protocols, including evacuation procedures, patient triage, and infection control measures.

Resource Management: Ensuring that there are adequate supplies, equipment, and personnel available during emergencies is essential. This includes having access to emergency medical supplies, power generators, and surge capacity plans.

Communication: Establishing effective communication systems is critical for coordinating response efforts. This includes both internal communication within the healthcare facility and external communication with emergency response agencies and the public.

Patient Care Continuity: Plans should be in place to ensure that patient care continues uninterrupted during emergencies, including providing care to patients with chronic conditions or those requiring life-sustaining treatments.

Drills and Exercises: Regular drills and exercises are essential to evaluate the preparedness of healthcare facilities and personnel. These simulations help identify strengths and weaknesses in emergency response plans.

Principles of Effective Response

Swift Action: The most critical element of emergency response is acting quickly to mitigate the impact of the event and save lives.

Flexibility: Response plans should be flexible and adaptable to evolving circumstances during an emergency.

Coordination: Effective coordination among healthcare facilities, first responders, public health agencies, and government entities is essential to ensure a cohesive response.

Safety First: The safety of patients and healthcare personnel should be the top priority. This includes ensuring the physical and psychological well-being of all involved.

Communication: Clear and concise communication is vital for sharing information, coordinating efforts, and providing guidance to the public.

Resource Management: Effective allocation and management of resources, including personnel, medical supplies, and transportation, are essential for a successful response.

Community Engagement: Involving the community in preparedness efforts and educating them about emergency plans and response expectations enhances overall resilience.

Saving Lives and Minimizing Harm

Emergency preparedness is a cornerstone of healthcare and public safety, focusing on proactive planning and readiness to respond effectively to emergencies. By following well-developed plans, training personnel, and maintaining critical resources, healthcare facilities can save lives, minimize harm, and contribute to the resilience of their communities during times of crisis.

Chapter 4:
Effective Communication

Therapeutic Communication: Building Trusting Patient Relationships

Therapeutic communication is a specialized form of communication that nurses use to establish and maintain a trusting and therapeutic relationship with patients. This communication style is essential because it not only helps in delivering quality patient care but also enhances the patient's overall experience and outcomes. Here's an explanation of therapeutic communication in nursing and its role in building trusting patient relationships:

Establishing Trust: Trust is the foundation of any nurse-patient relationship. Nurses must establish trust by being honest, reliable, and consistent in their care. Patients need to feel that they can rely on their nurses to meet their physical and emotional needs.

Active Listening: Nurses should actively listen to patients, giving them their full attention. This involves not only hearing the patient's words but also understanding their emotions and concerns. Active listening demonstrates that the nurse cares about the patient's well-being.

Empathy: Nurses should put themselves in the patient's shoes to understand their feelings and experiences. Demonstrating empathy shows patients that their nurse is compassionate and understanding of their physical and emotional pain or distress.

Nonverbal Communication: Nonverbal cues, such as eye contact, facial expressions, and body language, play a significant role in therapeutic communication. Maintaining appropriate eye contact and using body language that conveys warmth and empathy helps patients feel valued and understood.

Open and Honest Communication: Nurses should provide patients with accurate and honest information about their condition, treatment options, and progress. Open and honest communication builds trust and empowers patients to make informed decisions about their care.

Respect for Privacy and Dignity: Nurses should respect the patient's privacy and dignity at all times. This includes maintaining confidentiality and ensuring that the patient is comfortable and respected during physical examinations and procedures.

Patient-Centered Approach: Nursing care should be patient-centered, meaning it considers the patient's individual needs, preferences, and values. Nurses should involve patients in their care plans and decisions, fostering a sense of control and ownership over their health.

Cultural Sensitivity: Nurses must be culturally sensitive and aware of the diversity of patients they may encounter. Understanding and respecting cultural beliefs and practices are essential for effective communication and trust-building.

Education and Empowerment: Nurses should educate patients about their conditions, medications, and self-care strategies. Empowering patients with knowledge helps them take an active role in managing their health and promotes trust in the nurse's expertise.

Conflict Resolution: In situations where disagreements or conflicts arise, nurses should address them professionally and constructively. Conflict resolution skills are crucial in maintaining a positive nurse-patient relationship.

Continuity of Care: Consistency in nursing care builds trust. Patients feel more secure when they see the same nurse consistently involved in their care, providing continuity and a sense of familiarity.

Therapeutic communication in nursing is a holistic approach to interacting with patients that goes beyond simple information exchange. It involves establishing trust, active listening, empathy, and maintaining open, respectful, and patient-centered communication. When nurses employ therapeutic communication techniques, they can build trusting relationships with their patients, ultimately leading to better patient outcomes and overall satisfaction with their healthcare experiences.

Family-Centered Care: Engaging and Supporting Patients' Loved Ones

Family-centered care is an approach in nursing and healthcare that recognizes the importance of patients' families and loved ones as active participants in the patient's care and well-being. It involves engaging and supporting the patient's family in the healthcare process, as they can play a crucial role in the patient's recovery, comfort, and overall experience. Here's an explanation of family-centered care:

Inclusive Approach: Family-centered care acknowledges that patients' families are an integral part of their lives. It encourages healthcare providers to involve family members in care discussions, decision-making, and planning. This approach extends beyond the immediate family and can include anyone the patient considers significant to their well-being.

Communication and Collaboration: Nurses and healthcare teams should maintain open and effective communication with patients' families. This involves sharing information about the patient's condition, treatment options, and progress. Collaboration ensures that the family's insights and concerns are considered in the care plan.

Education and Support: Healthcare providers should offer education and support to patients' families. This includes explaining medical procedures, medications, and the patient's condition in understandable terms. Providing information helps families make informed decisions and cope with the challenges of caregiving.

Respect for Family Values: Family-centered care respects the cultural, religious, and personal values of the patient's family. This means accommodating their beliefs and preferences whenever possible, within the bounds of safe and effective care.

Emotional Support: Patients' families often experience emotional distress when their loved one is ill. Nurses can provide emotional support by actively listening to their concerns, offering counseling or resources, and being empathetic and compassionate.

Advocacy: Nurses can serve as advocates for both the patient and their family. They can ensure that the family's concerns are heard and addressed within the healthcare system. Advocacy helps empower families to be active participants in the patient's care.

Information Sharing: Keep the family updated on the patient's condition and progress. Transparency in communication builds trust and helps families understand what to expect during the healthcare journey.

Care Coordination: Family-centered care often involves coordinating care among different healthcare providers and services. Nurses can help facilitate this coordination to ensure that the patient receives comprehensive and consistent care.

Preparing Families for Transitions: When a patient is transitioning from one care setting to another (e.g., hospital to home), nurses can prepare families by providing information on how to care for the patient at home, including medication management and signs to watch for.

Supporting Decision-Making: Engage with families in making decisions about the patient's care, especially when there are complex treatment choices or end-of-life decisions to be made. Provide information and guidance while respecting the family's choices.

Feedback and Evaluation: Encourage feedback from families about their experiences with the healthcare team and the care provided. This input can lead to improvements in the quality of care and the family's overall experience.

Family-centered care recognizes that patients do not exist in isolation but are part of a larger support network. By engaging and supporting patients' loved ones, nurses can contribute to better patient outcomes, improved family satisfaction, and a more comprehensive and holistic approach to healthcare.

Interprofessional Collaboration: Working Effectively in Healthcare Teams

Interprofessional collaboration in healthcare refers to the practice of healthcare professionals from various disciplines working together as a team to provide comprehensive, patient-centered care. It recognizes that delivering quality healthcare requires the collective expertise and contributions of individuals with different skills and knowledge. Here's an explanation of interprofessional collaboration and its importance in healthcare:

Diverse Team Members: Interprofessional teams typically include professionals from various healthcare disciplines, such as physicians, nurses, pharmacists, physical therapists, social workers, and more. Each team member brings unique expertise and perspectives to the table.

Patient-Centered Care: The primary focus of interprofessional collaboration is the patient. It ensures that care is tailored to the individual's specific needs, preferences, and goals. This approach leads to more holistic and effective care.

Improved Health Outcomes: Research has shown that when healthcare professionals collaborate effectively, patients tend to experience better health outcomes. Coordinated care reduces errors, minimizes duplication of services, and enhances the overall quality of care.

Efficient Resource Utilization: Interprofessional collaboration optimizes the use of healthcare resources. It helps prevent unnecessary tests and treatments and ensures that patients receive the right care at the right time.

Enhanced Communication: Effective communication among team members is crucial in interprofessional collaboration. It involves sharing information, clarifying roles and responsibilities, and resolving conflicts. Clear communication helps prevent misunderstandings and errors.

Shared Decision-Making: Team members collaborate to make informed decisions about the patient's care. Shared decision-making involves discussing treatment options, risks, and benefits with the patient and their family, ensuring that their preferences and values are considered.

Continuity of Care: Interprofessional teams provide continuity of care as patients transition between different healthcare settings, such as from the hospital to a rehabilitation facility or home care. This seamless transition helps prevent gaps in care and reduces readmissions.

Education and Training: Interprofessional collaboration provides opportunities for team members to learn from each other and share their knowledge and skills. It contributes to ongoing professional development and a deeper understanding of each other's roles.

Increased Accountability: When healthcare professionals work collaboratively, there is a shared sense of responsibility for patient outcomes. This accountability motivates team members to provide the best possible care.

Addressing Complex Cases: Some medical conditions require the expertise of multiple specialists. Interprofessional collaboration allows healthcare teams to address complex cases more effectively, ensuring that patients receive comprehensive care.

Cost-Effective Care: By reducing redundancies and optimizing resource utilization, interprofessional collaboration can help control healthcare costs in the long run.

Patient and Family Involvement: Patients and their families are often included as active members of the healthcare team, especially in decisions about chronic disease management or end-of-life care.

Interprofessional collaboration is essential in healthcare because it harnesses the collective expertise of a diverse group of professionals to provide patient-centered, high-quality care. It promotes effective communication, shared decision-making, and the efficient use of resources, all of which lead to improved patient outcomes and a more satisfying healthcare experience for patients and their families.

Chapter 5:
Ethical Practice and Cultural Competence

Nursing Ethics: Navigating Complex Moral Issues

Nursing ethics is a branch of bioethics that deals with the ethical principles and dilemmas that nurses encounter in their practice. It provides a framework for nurses to navigate complex moral issues and make ethical decisions that prioritize the well-being and rights of patients. Here's an explanation of nursing ethics and how nurses navigate these complex moral issues:

Autonomy: One of the core principles of nursing ethics is respect for patient autonomy. Nurses must respect a patient's right to make informed decisions about their healthcare, even if those decisions differ from what the nurse believes is best. This includes obtaining informed consent for treatments and respecting the patient's right to refuse treatment.

Beneficence: Nurses have a duty to promote the well-being and best interests of their patients. This means providing care that is in the patient's best interest, striving to relieve suffering, and ensuring that patients receive the highest standard of care available.

Non-Maleficence: The principle of non-maleficence emphasizes that nurses must do no harm to patients. Nurses should avoid any actions that could harm patients and should always prioritize patient safety.

Justice: Justice in nursing ethics means treating patients fairly and equitably. Nurses must ensure that healthcare resources are distributed fairly, that care is accessible to all patients, and that they do not discriminate against patients based on factors like race, gender, or socioeconomic status.

Veracity: Veracity relates to honesty and truthfulness. Nurses have an ethical obligation to provide accurate information to patients and their families, including conveying the benefits and risks of treatments honestly and without deception.

Confidentiality: Nurses are bound by strict rules of confidentiality. They must protect the privacy of patients and ensure that their personal health information is not disclosed without their consent, except in cases where it is required by law or necessary for patient care.

Fidelity: Fidelity involves being faithful and loyal to patients. Nurses must uphold their professional responsibilities and commitments to patients, including providing care with competence, integrity, and honesty.

Nurses often encounter complex moral issues in their practice, such as:

End-of-life care: Decisions about withholding or withdrawing life-sustaining treatment, Do-Not-Resuscitate (DNR) orders, and advance care planning can raise ethical dilemmas.

Resource allocation: Nurses may face ethical challenges related to allocating limited healthcare resources, such as ventilators or organ transplants, in situations of high demand.

Conflicts of interest: Nurses may encounter conflicts of interest that require them to balance their professional obligations with personal or financial interests.

Cultural and religious beliefs: Differences in cultural and religious beliefs between nurses and patients can lead to ethical dilemmas, such as decisions about blood transfusions or end-of-life rituals.

To navigate these complex moral issues, nurses often engage in ethical decision-making processes that involve assessing the situation, identifying ethical principles at stake, consulting with colleagues and ethics committees, and making decisions that are consistent with ethical standards and the best interests of the patient.

Nursing ethics provides a moral compass for nurses, guiding them in delivering care that respects the dignity, autonomy, and rights of patients while upholding the highest ethical standards of the profession.

Legal Aspects of Nursing: Understanding the Legal Framework

Understanding the legal aspects of nursing is essential for nurses to provide safe and ethical care while protecting both their patients and themselves. The legal framework governing nursing practice varies by country and state, but it generally covers a range of topics. Here's an overview of the key elements of the legal aspects of nursing:

Nursing Practice Acts and Regulations: Nursing practice is typically governed by state-specific Nursing Practice Acts and regulations. These laws define the scope of practice for nurses, outlining the tasks and responsibilities they are allowed to perform. It's crucial for nurses to be familiar with the Nursing Practice Act in their state.

Licensure: Nurses must obtain and maintain a valid nursing license to practice legally. Licensure requirements, including education, examinations, and renewal processes, are determined by the state nursing board.

Scope of Practice: Each category of nursing (e.g., registered nurse, licensed practical nurse) has a defined scope of practice. Nurses must adhere to their specific scope and not engage in activities outside of it. Violating the scope of practice can lead to legal consequences.

Standards of Care: Nurses are expected to provide care that meets established standards of practice. Deviating from these standards can result in legal liability if patient harm occurs.

Patient Rights and Informed Consent: Nurses must respect and protect patients' rights, including the right to informed consent. This involves ensuring patients understand the risks and benefits of treatments and procedures before providing their consent.

Documentation: Accurate and timely documentation of patient care is crucial. Nurses should maintain clear, complete, and legally sound records. Good documentation can be vital in legal cases, helping to establish the care provided and the patient's condition.

Confidentiality: Nurses are bound by laws and ethical standards to maintain patient confidentiality. Disclosing patient information without consent can lead to legal and ethical violations.

Malpractice and Negligence: Malpractice occurs when a healthcare professional fails to provide care that meets established standards, resulting in patient harm. Negligence is a component of malpractice and involves the failure to exercise reasonable care. Nurses can be held legally liable for malpractice and negligence.

Duty of Care: Nurses have a legal duty to provide care to the best of their abilities. This duty exists once a nurse-patient relationship is established, and it continues until care is appropriately transferred or terminated.

Reporting Requirements: Nurses often have legal obligations to report certain situations, such as suspected child abuse, elder abuse, or infectious diseases, to the appropriate authorities.

Advance Directives and End-of-Life Care: Nurses may be involved in decisions related to advance directives, do-not-resuscitate (DNR) orders, and end-of-life care. Understanding the legal aspects of these issues is crucial to ensure compliance with patient wishes and legal requirements.

Employment Contracts: Nurses should carefully review and understand their employment contracts, which may contain specific legal obligations and responsibilities related to their position.

Continuing Education: Many states require nurses to complete continuing education to maintain their licensure. Understanding and complying with these requirements is essential.

Legal Protections: Nurses may have legal protections, such as whistleblower laws, that shield them from retaliation when reporting unsafe or unethical practices in their workplace.

Nurses must stay up-to-date with changes in nursing laws and regulations and seek legal counsel when facing complex legal issues. Being knowledgeable about the legal framework of nursing practice is essential for providing high-quality, safe, and ethical care while minimizing legal risks.

Cultural Competence: Providing Culturally Sensitive Care

Cultural competence is the ability to provide care that is respectful, sensitive, and responsive to the cultural beliefs, values, practices, and needs of patients and their families. It is an essential aspect of nursing practice, as it helps to bridge cultural gaps, reduce health disparities, and ensure that healthcare is delivered in a way that respects the diversity of the patient population. Here's an explanation of cultural competence in nursing and its importance:

Understanding Cultural Diversity: Cultural competence starts with an understanding and appreciation of the cultural diversity that exists among patients. This includes recognizing that culture encompasses not only race and ethnicity but also religion, language, socioeconomic status, gender, sexual orientation, and more.

Avoiding Stereotypes and Assumptions: Nurses must avoid making assumptions or relying on stereotypes about patients based on their cultural background. Every patient is an individual with unique beliefs and preferences.

Active Listening: Cultural competence involves active listening to patients and their families. This means giving them the opportunity to share their cultural beliefs and values as they relate to their healthcare. It also means paying attention to nonverbal cues and body language, which can convey important cultural information.

Respect for Cultural Practices: Nurses should respect and accommodate cultural practices and preferences that do not conflict with safe and effective care. This might include dietary restrictions, preferred methods of communication, or religious practices.

Language Competence: When language barriers exist, nurses should make efforts to ensure effective communication. This may involve using professional interpreters or utilizing translation services to convey medical information accurately.

Culturally Sensitive Assessments: Nurses should adapt their assessment techniques to be culturally sensitive. For example, understanding that some cultures may have different expressions of pain or may be hesitant to discuss certain health issues openly.

Cultural Awareness of Health Beliefs: Understanding the cultural beliefs about health and illness is crucial. Some cultures may have traditional healing practices or alternative therapies that should be considered in conjunction with Western medicine.

Cultural Humility: Cultural competence also involves cultural humility, which is an ongoing process of self-reflection and self-awareness regarding one's own cultural biases and limitations. It means recognizing that you may not know everything about a particular culture and being open to learning from your patients.

Inclusivity: Ensure that healthcare settings are inclusive and welcoming to individuals from diverse backgrounds. This includes the physical environment, literature, and the staff's cultural sensitivity.

Collaboration: Collaborate with interdisciplinary teams that include cultural experts, interpreters, and social workers when necessary to provide the most appropriate and sensitive care.

Patient-Centered Care: Always prioritize patient-centered care, which means involving the patient in decision-making and tailoring care plans to align with their cultural values and preferences.

Cultural competence is important because it not only respects patients' rights to receive care that aligns with their cultural beliefs but also leads to better patient outcomes. When patients feel understood and respected in healthcare settings, they are more likely to trust their healthcare providers, adhere to treatment plans, and engage in preventive care. Cultural competence is not a static skill but a lifelong learning process that is essential for providing high-quality, patient-centered care in a diverse and multicultural society.

Chapter 6:
Education and Patient Advocacy

Patient Education: Empowering Patients for Self-Care

Patient education is a vital component of nursing care that aims to empower patients with the knowledge and skills they need to actively participate in their own healthcare and make informed decisions. This process helps patients take ownership of their health and enhances their ability to engage in self-care. Here's an explanation of patient education in nursing and its importance:

Assessment: The first step in patient education is assessing the patient's current level of knowledge, health literacy, and learning needs. Nurses need to understand what the patient already knows and what information or skills they require to manage their health effectively.

Clear Communication: Effective communication is key to patient education. Nurses should use clear, simple language and avoid medical jargon to ensure that the patient can understand the information being conveyed.

Individualized Education: Patient education should be tailored to each patient's specific needs, preferences, and cultural background. What works for one patient may not work for another, so a personalized approach is essential.

Setting Realistic Goals: Collaboratively establish goals with the patient. These goals should be specific, measurable, achievable, relevant, and time-bound (SMART). This helps patients track their progress and stay motivated.

Use of Visual Aids: Visual aids, such as diagrams, charts, and videos, can be invaluable in patient education. They can help patients grasp complex concepts and instructions more easily.

Repetition: Patients may need information repeated multiple times for it to sink in. Nurses should be patient and willing to provide reinforcement when necessary.

Engagement: Encourage patients to ask questions and be actively involved in their learning process. Actively involving patients fosters a sense of ownership over their health.

Medication Education: Ensure that patients understand their medications, including dosages, administration methods, and potential side effects. Non-adherence to medication regimens can lead to health complications.

Lifestyle Modification: Educate patients about healthy lifestyle choices, including nutrition, exercise, and stress management. Provide practical tips for making sustainable changes.

Prevention: Emphasize preventive healthcare measures, such as immunizations and regular screenings, to help patients maintain good health and catch potential issues early.

Chronic Disease Management: For patients with chronic conditions, provide comprehensive education on disease management, including symptom recognition, monitoring, and strategies for managing flare-ups.

Safety Measures: Educate patients on safety precautions, such as fall prevention and infection control, to minimize risks during their healthcare journey.

Community Resources: Inform patients about available community resources and support groups that can complement their self-care efforts.

Technology: In today's digital age, nurses may also educate patients on how to use healthcare technology, such as health apps or telemedicine services, to manage their health effectively.

Documentation: Properly document patient education efforts in the patient's health record to track what has been covered, ensure continuity of care, and demonstrate compliance with regulatory requirements.

Patient education is a collaborative process that empowers patients to actively participate in their healthcare decisions and improve their health outcomes. It is not a one-time event but an ongoing process that should be integrated into every patient interaction to promote self-care, prevent complications, and enhance the patient's overall well-being.

Palliative and End-of-Life Care: Ensuring Comfort and Dignity

Palliative and end-of-life care in nursing is a specialized area of healthcare focused on providing comfort, support, and dignity to patients who are facing life-limiting illnesses, as well as their families. The goal is to enhance the quality of life, relieve suffering, and ensure that patients experience a peaceful and dignified transition at the end of life. Here's an explanation of palliative and end-of-life care:

Palliative Care vs. Hospice Care: Palliative care is an approach that can be integrated at any stage of a serious illness, not just at the end of life. It focuses on managing symptoms, improving the patient's quality of life, and addressing the emotional and psychological aspects of illness. Hospice care, on the other hand, is a type of palliative care specifically designed for patients with a prognosis of six months or less to live. It is typically initiated when curative treatments are no longer effective.

Pain and Symptom Management: Effective pain and symptom management is a cornerstone of palliative care. Nurses play a critical role in assessing and addressing pain, discomfort, and distressing symptoms, such as nausea, shortness of breath, and anxiety. Medication management is often a key aspect of this care.

Holistic Assessment: Nurses conduct comprehensive assessments that go beyond physical symptoms. They consider the patient's psychological, social, and spiritual needs. This holistic approach helps nurses provide well-rounded care that addresses all aspects of the patient's well-being.

Advance Care Planning: Nurses assist patients and families in making informed decisions about their care preferences, including advance directives, resuscitation preferences, and goals of care. These discussions help ensure that the patient's wishes are respected.

Emotional and Psychological Support: Patients and families facing end-of-life issues often experience emotional distress. Nurses offer emotional support by actively listening, providing a safe space for expression, and connecting patients and families with counselors or support groups.

Cultural Sensitivity: Understanding and respecting the cultural, religious, and spiritual beliefs and practices of patients and families is crucial in end-of-life care. This sensitivity ensures that care aligns with the patient's values and preferences.

Communication: Effective communication is essential in palliative and end-of-life care. Nurses facilitate discussions between the patient, family, and healthcare team, ensuring that everyone is on the same page regarding the care plan and goals.

Comfort Measures: Nurses provide comfort measures that go beyond medical interventions. This may include creating a calming environment, offering gentle touch, or helping patients with activities they find meaningful.

Family Support: Supporting the patient's family is an integral part of end-of-life care. Nurses provide guidance, education, and emotional support to help families cope with the impending loss of a loved one.

Ethical Issues: Nurses may encounter complex ethical dilemmas, such as decisions about withholding or withdrawing life-sustaining treatment. They must navigate these issues while upholding ethical principles and ensuring that the patient's best interests are at the forefront.

Dignity and Respect: Above all, nurses work to ensure that patients experience a dignified and peaceful transition. This includes preserving the patient's autonomy, privacy, and comfort.

Grief Support: After a patient's passing, nurses continue to support the family through the grieving process, offering resources and referrals to bereavement services.

Palliative and end-of-life care in nursing is emotionally demanding but incredibly rewarding. It allows nurses to make a profound difference in the lives of patients and their families during a vulnerable and challenging time. The focus on comfort, dignity, and holistic care ensures that individuals facing life-limiting illnesses can experience the best possible quality of life until the end.

Healthcare Quality Improvement: Implementing Evidence-Based Practice

Healthcare quality improvement in nursing involves the systematic approach to enhancing the safety, effectiveness, and overall quality of patient care. One key aspect of quality improvement is the implementation of evidence-based practice (EBP). EBP involves integrating the best available research evidence, clinical expertise, and patient preferences to guide nursing care decisions. Here's an explanation of healthcare quality improvement through implementing evidence-based practice in nursing:

Evaluating Current Practices: The first step in quality improvement is to assess current nursing practices and identify areas that may benefit from changes or updates. This might involve reviewing clinical processes, patient outcomes, and feedback from patients and healthcare teams.

Identifying Evidence: EBP relies on the best available evidence from research studies, clinical guidelines, and other credible sources. Nurses must stay up-to-date with the latest research findings to inform their practice.

Clinical Expertise: Nurses bring their own clinical expertise and experience to the table. EBP involves integrating this knowledge with research evidence to make well-informed decisions that are appropriate for individual patients.

Patient Preferences and Values: Patient-centered care considers the preferences, values, and goals of patients in decision-making. Nurses should engage patients in discussions about their care options and involve them in the decision-making process.

Developing Protocols and Guidelines: Based on the evidence, clinical expertise, and patient preferences, nursing protocols, and guidelines can be developed or updated. These protocols provide a standardized approach to care that reflects the best available evidence.

Multidisciplinary Collaboration: Quality improvement often involves collaboration among healthcare professionals from various disciplines. Nurses work alongside physicians, pharmacists, therapists, and other team members to implement evidence-based practices and ensure consistent care.

Pilot Testing: Before implementing changes across a healthcare setting, nurses may pilot test new protocols or interventions in a controlled environment. This allows for adjustments and fine-tuning before broader implementation.

Monitoring and Data Collection: Quality improvement relies on data collection to measure the impact of changes. Nurses use data to track patient outcomes, adherence to protocols, and any variations in practice.

Continuous Evaluation: Quality improvement is an ongoing process. Nurses regularly evaluate the effectiveness of changes and gather feedback from patients and colleagues to make further refinements if necessary.

Education and Training: Implementing EBP often requires educating and training nursing staff about the new protocols or practices. This ensures that all members of the team are on the same page.

Barriers and Challenges: Nurses need to be aware of potential barriers to implementing EBP, such as resistance to change, resource constraints, or lack of time. Addressing these challenges is an important part of the quality improvement process.

Leadership Support: Leadership within healthcare organizations plays a crucial role in supporting and promoting EBP initiatives. Nursing leaders can allocate resources, encourage staff participation, and foster a culture of continuous improvement.

Dissemination of Findings: When evidence-based practices lead to positive outcomes, nurses can share their findings with the broader healthcare community through presentations, publications, or conferences.

Implementing evidence-based practice in nursing contributes to safer, more effective, and patient-centered care. By combining the best available evidence with clinical expertise and patient preferences, nurses can ensure that their practice is both informed and continuously improving, ultimately leading to better patient outcomes and overall healthcare quality.

Chapter 7:
Leadership and Management

Leadership in Nursing: Influencing Positive Change

Leadership in nursing is about guiding, inspiring, and influencing positive change within the healthcare system and among nursing teams. Effective nursing leaders play a critical role in shaping the quality of patient care, fostering a positive work environment, and driving improvements in healthcare delivery. Here's an explanation of leadership in nursing and its role in influencing positive change:

Vision and Purpose: Nursing leaders articulate a clear vision and purpose that align with the organization's mission and values. This vision provides direction and motivation for nursing teams.

Clinical Expertise: Effective nursing leaders are knowledgeable and skilled in clinical practice. They earn the respect and trust of their teams by demonstrating competence and staying up-to-date with best practices.

Collaboration: Nursing leaders foster a culture of collaboration, encouraging multidisciplinary teamwork and communication. Collaborative approaches lead to improved patient outcomes and a more positive work environment.

Advocacy: Advocacy for patients, staff, and the nursing profession is a crucial aspect of nursing leadership. Leaders ensure that patient rights are respected, staff have the resources they need, and nursing practice is evidence-based.

Change Management: Healthcare is constantly evolving, and nursing leaders play a pivotal role in managing change effectively. They help staff adapt to new technologies, procedures, or policies and navigate the challenges that come with change.

Inspiration and Motivation: Effective nursing leaders inspire and motivate their teams to excel. They recognize and celebrate achievements and provide encouragement during difficult times.

Problem-Solving: Nursing leaders are adept at identifying and solving problems. They use critical thinking skills to address challenges in patient care, workflow, or resource allocation.

Ethical Decision-Making: Ethical decision-making is a fundamental aspect of nursing leadership. Leaders uphold ethical principles and guide their teams in making morally sound choices.

Mentorship and Development: Nursing leaders support the professional growth and development of their staff. They mentor and coach emerging leaders and provide opportunities for continuing education.

Quality Improvement: Leaders champion quality improvement initiatives that enhance patient care and safety. They use data-driven approaches to identify areas for improvement and implement evidence-based practices.

Resource Management: Nursing leaders are responsible for efficiently managing resources, including staffing, budgets, and equipment, to ensure that patient care needs are met.

Adaptability: Effective nursing leaders are adaptable and flexible in the face of challenges or unexpected events. They remain calm and make informed decisions under pressure.

Advocacy for Staff: Nursing leaders advocate for their staff's needs, well-being, and work-life balance. They promote a healthy work environment that prevents burnout and turnover.

Continuous Learning: Leadership in nursing involves continuous learning and self-improvement. Leaders stay informed about healthcare trends, leadership theories, and management strategies.

Feedback and Evaluation: Leaders provide constructive feedback to staff and conduct regular performance evaluations. This feedback loop helps identify areas for improvement and development.

Leadership in nursing is a multifaceted role that involves guiding and inspiring nursing teams to provide high-quality patient care and drive positive change in healthcare. Effective nursing leaders possess a combination of clinical expertise, communication skills, and the ability to foster collaboration and continuous improvement. They are instrumental in creating a culture of excellence, ensuring patient safety, and advancing the nursing profession.

Healthcare Management: Navigating Administrative Roles

Healthcare management in nursing involves assuming administrative roles and responsibilities within healthcare organizations to ensure efficient and effective delivery of patient care services. Nurse managers, directors of nursing, and other administrative nursing roles play a crucial role in overseeing operations, managing resources, and ensuring quality care. Here's an explanation of healthcare management in nursing and the key aspects of navigating administrative roles:

Leadership and Administration: Administrative nurses are leaders who set the tone for their departments or units. They provide direction, make decisions, and motivate staff to achieve organizational goals.

Resource Allocation: Healthcare managers are responsible for managing resources effectively, including budgets, staffing, equipment, and supplies. They must balance resource availability with the need to provide high-quality care.

Staffing and Scheduling: Nurse managers oversee staffing levels and scheduling to ensure that patient needs are met while maintaining a safe and manageable workload for the nursing staff. This involves making decisions about hiring, training, and scheduling.

Quality Improvement: Healthcare administrators work to enhance the quality of patient care. They implement quality improvement initiatives, monitor outcomes, and use data to drive continuous improvement efforts.

Regulatory Compliance: Nursing leaders are responsible for ensuring that their units or departments comply with healthcare regulations and standards, including those related to patient safety, documentation, and accreditation.

Performance Evaluation: Nurse managers conduct performance evaluations for their staff, providing feedback and guidance to improve individual and team performance.

Communication: Effective communication is essential for healthcare managers. They must convey organizational goals and expectations to their teams, as well as relay information from upper management to frontline staff.

Patient-Centered Care: Healthcare administrators prioritize patient-centered care, ensuring that patient needs and preferences are at the forefront of decision-making and service delivery.

Conflict Resolution: Nursing leaders often mediate conflicts among staff members, helping to maintain a harmonious work environment. Conflict resolution skills are crucial for addressing personnel issues.

Strategic Planning: Administrative nurses participate in strategic planning for their units or departments. They align their goals and activities with the broader organizational mission and vision.

Budget Management: Nurse managers are responsible for developing and managing budgets. This includes allocating resources, controlling costs, and ensuring that financial goals are met.

Continuing Education: Staying up-to-date with healthcare trends, regulations, and management practices is essential for healthcare administrators. They often engage in continuing education to enhance their leadership skills.

Technology Utilization: Administrative nurses leverage healthcare technology and electronic health records to streamline processes, improve documentation, and enhance patient care.

Patient and Family Engagement: Nurse managers may implement strategies to involve patients and families in care decisions and improvement efforts, recognizing their valuable insights.

Emergency Preparedness: Nurse managers ensure that their units are prepared to respond effectively to emergencies and disasters, with well-defined protocols and training in place.

Navigating administrative roles in nursing requires a blend of leadership skills, healthcare knowledge, and management expertise. Effective healthcare managers are instrumental in optimizing patient care, ensuring regulatory compliance, and contributing to the overall success of healthcare organizations.

Professional Development: Advancing Your Nursing Career

Professional development in nursing refers to the continuous process of acquiring new knowledge, skills, and competencies to enhance one's nursing practice, advance their career, and provide the highest quality of care to patients. It involves a commitment to lifelong learning, self-improvement, and staying up-to-date with the latest advancements in healthcare. Here's an explanation of professional development in nursing and its importance for advancing your nursing career:

Continuing Education: Professional development often involves pursuing additional education beyond the initial nursing degree. This could include attending workshops, seminars, conferences, and online courses to deepen your understanding of specific nursing topics or acquire new skills.

Specialty Certification: Obtaining specialty certifications in areas such as critical care, pediatrics, oncology, or geriatrics demonstrates your expertise in a particular nursing field. Certification enhances your credibility and opens up opportunities for career advancement.

Advanced Degrees: Pursuing advanced degrees, such as a Master of Science in Nursing (MSN) or a Doctor of Nursing Practice (DNP), can lead to more specialized roles, such as nurse practitioner, nurse educator, or nurse leader.

Skill Enhancement: Professional development allows you to acquire and refine clinical and non-clinical skills, such as leadership, communication, critical thinking, and technology proficiency.

Evidence-Based Practice: Staying current with evidence-based practice is essential for providing the best possible patient care. Professional development enables you to incorporate the latest research and best practices into your nursing care.

Networking: Participating in professional organizations, conferences, and workshops provides opportunities to network with fellow nurses, share experiences, and learn from others in the field.

Leadership Development: Professional development can prepare you for leadership roles by enhancing your management skills, conflict resolution abilities, and decision-making capabilities.

Teaching and Education: For nurses interested in education, professional development can provide the skills and knowledge needed to become effective nurse educators, teaching the next generation of nurses.

Career Advancement: Professional development often leads to expanded career opportunities. Acquiring new skills and certifications can position you for promotions, higher-paying positions, and roles with greater responsibility.

Personal Fulfillment: Engaging in professional development can be personally fulfilling as you gain a sense of accomplishment and confidence in your abilities. It can lead to increased job satisfaction and a greater sense of purpose in your nursing career.

Adapting to Change: Healthcare is constantly evolving, with new technologies, treatments, and regulations. Professional development helps you stay adaptable and ready to embrace changes in the field.

Patient Safety: Updated knowledge and skills gained through professional development directly contribute to patient safety by ensuring that you provide the most current and evidence-based care.

Ethical Practice: Professional development can enhance your understanding of ethical dilemmas and provide you with tools to navigate complex situations while upholding ethical principles.

Continual Improvement: Committing to professional development reflects your dedication to continual improvement and growth as a healthcare professional.

In today's rapidly changing healthcare landscape, ongoing professional development is essential for nurses to remain competent, adaptable, and at the forefront of their field. Whether you're seeking to expand your clinical expertise, pursue leadership roles, or contribute to healthcare education, investing in your professional development is a critical step toward advancing your nursing career and ensuring the highest quality of patient care.

Chapter 8:
Safety and Regulation

Patient Safety: Preventing Errors and Adverse Events

Patient safety in nursing is the proactive and systematic effort to prevent errors, reduce risks, and minimize harm to patients during their healthcare journey. It involves creating a culture of safety, implementing best practices, and fostering an environment where all healthcare team members prioritize patient well-being. Here's an explanation of patient safety in nursing and the measures taken to prevent errors and adverse events:

Culture of Safety: Creating a culture of safety is foundational to patient safety efforts. This involves promoting open communication, encouraging reporting of errors and near-misses without fear of retribution, and valuing teamwork and collaboration.

Effective Communication: Clear and accurate communication among healthcare team members is essential for preventing errors. Nurses must communicate vital information, such as patient allergies, medications, and treatment plans, accurately and promptly.

Medication Safety: Nurses play a critical role in medication administration. This includes verifying patient identities, checking medication labels, administering the correct dose, and documenting accurately. Using barcode scanning technology and performing "five rights" checks (right patient, right medication, right dose, right route, right time) can prevent medication errors.

Patient Identification: Ensuring accurate patient identification using two patient identifiers (e.g., name and date of birth) helps prevent errors related to incorrect patient data.

Hand Hygiene: Proper hand hygiene is a simple yet effective measure to prevent the spread of infections, protecting both patients and healthcare workers.

Infection Prevention: Following infection prevention protocols, such as maintaining a clean environment, using appropriate personal protective equipment (PPE), and adhering to isolation precautions, prevents healthcare-associated infections.

Fall Prevention: Assessing patient fall risk and implementing fall prevention measures, such as using bed alarms, providing non-slip footwear, and assisting patients with mobility, helps prevent falls and related injuries.

Surgical Safety: Nurses collaborate with surgical teams to ensure correct surgical site identification, proper preoperative assessments, accurate surgical instrument counts, and compliance with safety checklists.

Documentation Accuracy: Accurate and thorough documentation is crucial for patient safety. Nurses should document interventions, assessments, and patient responses accurately to provide a clear record of care.

Patient Education: Educating patients about their conditions, medications, treatments, and self-care measures empowers them to actively participate in their own safety.

Safe Staffing: Adequate staffing levels are essential to ensure that nurses can provide safe and effective care without being overwhelmed by high patient loads.

Evidence-Based Practice: Implementing evidence-based practices and adhering to clinical guidelines ensures that care is based on the best available research and reduces the risk of errors.

Root Cause Analysis: When errors or adverse events occur, conducting root cause analysis helps identify underlying causes and implement corrective actions to prevent similar incidents in the future.

Simulation and Training: Using simulation and hands-on training allows nurses to practice high-risk situations in a controlled environment, enhancing their skills and confidence.

Reporting Systems: Encouraging nurses to report errors and near-misses through incident reporting systems helps identify potential risks and implement corrective actions.

Continuous Learning: Staying up-to-date with new healthcare technologies, procedures, and safety practices through ongoing education is essential for maintaining a high standard of patient safety.

Patient safety is a shared responsibility among all healthcare team members, with nurses playing a central role in preventing errors and adverse events. By promoting a culture of safety, adhering to best practices, and advocating for patient well-being, nurses contribute to providing high-quality care while minimizing the risk of harm to patients.

Regulatory Compliance: Upholding Nursing Standards

Regulatory compliance in nursing refers to the adherence to laws, regulations, and standards that govern nursing practice, patient care, and healthcare facilities. Upholding nursing standards through regulatory compliance is essential for ensuring patient safety, maintaining the quality of care, and promoting ethical nursing practice. Here's an explanation of regulatory compliance in nursing and its importance:

Licensure: Nurses are required to obtain and maintain a valid nursing license issued by the state nursing board in the jurisdiction where they practice. Regulatory compliance starts with ensuring that one's nursing license is up-to-date and in good standing.

Nursing Practice Acts: Nursing practice is regulated by state-specific Nursing Practice Acts. These laws define the scope of practice for nurses in a particular state, outlining what nurses can and cannot do. Compliance with the Nursing Practice Act is fundamental to legal nursing practice.

Accreditation and Certification: Healthcare facilities, including hospitals and clinics, often require accreditation from accrediting bodies like The Joint Commission. Nurses must adhere to the standards set forth by these organizations to ensure the facility remains compliant.

Documentation: Accurate and timely documentation of patient care is crucial for regulatory compliance. Nurses must maintain clear, complete, and legally sound records of patient assessments, interventions, and outcomes.

Medication Safety: Nurses are responsible for complying with medication safety standards, including verifying medication orders, administering medications accurately, and monitoring for adverse reactions.

Infection Control: Following infection control practices and guidelines is essential for preventing healthcare-associated infections. Nurses must adhere to hand hygiene protocols, use appropriate personal protective equipment (PPE), and follow isolation precautions.

Ethical Standards: Nurses are bound by ethical standards set by professional organizations like the American Nurses Association (ANA). These standards guide ethical nursing practice, emphasizing principles such as patient advocacy, confidentiality, and informed consent.

Patient Rights: Nurses must uphold patient rights, including the right to informed consent, privacy, and dignity. Understanding and respecting these rights are essential components of regulatory compliance.

HIPAA Compliance: The Health Insurance Portability and Accountability Act (HIPAA) governs the privacy and security of patient health information. Nurses must ensure that patient information is protected and only shared as allowed by law.

Continuing Education: Many states require nurses to complete continuing education as a condition of licensure renewal. Compliance with these education requirements ensures that nurses stay current with advances in healthcare practice.

Adherence to Protocols: Healthcare facilities often have protocols and policies in place to guide care delivery. Nurses must comply with these protocols to maintain consistency and quality of care.

Patient Safety Initiatives: Nurses should actively participate in patient safety initiatives within their healthcare organizations. This includes reporting safety concerns, near-misses, and adverse events to ensure a culture of safety.

Compliance with National Standards: Nurses are often expected to follow national nursing standards and guidelines, such as those published by the ANA or specialty-specific organizations like the Oncology Nursing Society or the Emergency Nurses Association.

Regulatory Reporting: In some cases, nurses may be required to report certain incidents or issues to regulatory bodies or state agencies, such as suspected abuse or violations of ethical standards.

Conflict Resolution: Nurses should be prepared to navigate conflicts or ethical dilemmas in a manner consistent with ethical standards and organizational policies.

Upholding nursing standards through regulatory compliance is essential for maintaining patient trust, ensuring safe and effective care, and protecting the integrity of the nursing profession. Failure to comply with regulations and standards can result in legal consequences and disciplinary actions against a nurse's license. Therefore, nurses must remain informed about relevant laws and regulations and make compliance a top priority in their practice.

Conclusion: Mastering Nursing Essentials

Embracing Lifelong Learning: Thriving as a Competent Nurse

Embracing lifelong learning is a core principle for nursing professionals who aim to thrive in their careers and remain competent in an ever-evolving healthcare landscape. Nursing is a dynamic field that continually advances with new technologies, treatments, and research findings. Here's an explanation of why lifelong learning is crucial for nurses and how it supports competence and growth:

Continuous Knowledge Expansion: Lifelong learning ensures that nurses stay current with the latest medical advancements, evidence-based practices, and treatment modalities. This knowledge expansion is essential for providing safe and effective patient care.

Adapting to Change: Healthcare is constantly changing, with new diseases, treatments, and technologies emerging regularly. Lifelong learners are better equipped to adapt to these changes and provide optimal care to patients.

Evidence-Based Practice: Lifelong learning enables nurses to integrate the best available evidence into their practice. This approach improves patient outcomes and ensures that care is aligned with the latest research.

Improved Patient Care: Competent nurses who engage in lifelong learning are more likely to provide high-quality, patient-centered care. Patients benefit from healthcare professionals who are knowledgeable and up-to-date.

Career Advancement: Lifelong learning opens up opportunities for career advancement, including promotions, leadership roles, and specialization in various nursing fields.

Professional Growth: Engaging in ongoing education and development fosters professional growth and job satisfaction. It allows nurses to take on new challenges and expand their horizons within the field.

Critical Thinking Skills: Lifelong learning enhances critical thinking and problem-solving abilities, which are essential for assessing complex patient situations and making informed decisions.

Ethical Decision-Making: Lifelong learners are better equipped to navigate ethical dilemmas and make decisions that align with ethical principles, ensuring patient safety and ethical practice.

Communication Skills: Nursing practice often involves complex communication with patients, families, and healthcare teams. Lifelong learning can improve interpersonal and communication skills, leading to better patient experiences.

Multidisciplinary Collaboration: Healthcare is delivered by a multidisciplinary team. Lifelong learners can collaborate effectively with physicians, therapists, social workers, and other healthcare professionals to ensure holistic care for patients.

Innovation: Lifelong learners are more likely to embrace innovative practices and technologies that can enhance patient care and streamline clinical processes.

Personal Fulfillment: Learning new skills and gaining knowledge can be personally fulfilling. Lifelong learners often experience a sense of accomplishment and fulfillment in their nursing careers.

Patient Safety: Lifelong learning contributes to patient safety by reducing the risk of errors and adverse events through the application of current best practices.

Role Model for Others: Nurses who prioritize lifelong learning serve as role models for their colleagues and future generations of nurses, inspiring a culture of continuous improvement in healthcare.

Professional Networking: Engaging in lifelong learning often involves networking with colleagues, educators, and experts in the field, providing opportunities to exchange knowledge and experiences.

To embrace lifelong learning as a competent nurse, individuals can pursue various avenues, including formal education, online courses, workshops, conferences, certifications, and professional organizations. Additionally, maintaining a curious and inquisitive mindset, seeking out opportunities for mentorship and collaboration, and reflecting on one's practice are essential aspects of lifelong learning. By committing to ongoing education and professional development, nurses can thrive in their careers, provide the best possible care to their patients, and make a meaningful impact on the nursing profession and healthcare as a whole.

- THE END -